ELIMINATION

GET OUT OF MY BODY!

A short and comprehensive handbook on the blood purification by elimination treatment for the beginners to the medical studies

I, as the author, assume all information in this book is believed to be true and accurate at the date of writing. The author does not give a warranty, express or implied, concerning the information contained herein or for any mistakes or omissions that he has made.

This work is not under any circumstances intended to be, and should not be considered, a substitute for any health or any different medical or other advice. Therapy for the conditions described in this material is highly dependent on individual patient conditions. As this work of mine is meant to offer accurate information with respect to the subject enclosed and to be current as of the time it was written, exploration and data about medical and health matters are continually evolving and dose schedules for medications are being revised continually, with new side effects recognized and accounted for on a regular basis. Readers of this book must therefore always read any medical or pharmaceutical product communication and clinical processes with the most up-to-date published product information and data sheets provided by the manufacturers of the products, summary of the product's characteristics and the most recent codes of conduct and safety regulation. The author of this book makes no representations or warranties to anybody, express or implied, as for the correctness or completeness of this communication provided. Without limiting the preceding, the author is not liable to accept, and particularly disclaim, any obligation for any liability, loss or risk that may be claimed or incurred because of the appropriate or inappropriate use and application of any of the content of this work.

The statements, opinions, and data contained in this book are those of the individual authors cited. The author has exerted every reasonable effort to ensure that drug selection and dosage outlined in this book of mine are in accord with current recommendations, guidelines, and practice at the time of writing. However, having current progress because of ongoing research, changes in various government regulations and the constant flow of information relating to any therapy and adverse reactions, the readers of this book are urged to check the package inserts for each drug for any change in indications and dosage and added warning and precautions. The measure is critical when the recommended agent is a new one and infrequently used.

This topic in more detail and like you can find in my publications from my Kidney Replacement series published on Amazon – Kindle Direct Publishing, e.g.,

BLOOD PURIFICATION

Specialized Work

By

Lubomir POLASCIN, MD

On

EXTRACORPOREAL ELIMINATION TREATMENT

Dialysis interventions to achieve required blood composition changes in men by its artificial machine purification on the principles of diffusion/dialysis, convection (membrane filtration), adsorption and osmosis.

KEYWORDS

acetate, acetic, acid acute hepatic failure, acute liver failure, adsorbers, adsorption, , albumin, ALF, arterial, arterialization, arterial-venous, artificial detoxification, autoimmune disease, autologous graft, back-diffusion, back-filtration, bicarbonate, bioartificial liver, biocomponent, biofunctional hepatic system, biofunctional liver system, biologic liver, support, bioreactor, blood, blood purification, catheter, catheters, chemical principles, cholesterol, circuit, circulation, citrate, citric acid, clearance, complications, concentration, continuous renal replacement therapy, convection, copolymers, CRRT, dialysate, dialysis, dialysis, dialysis device, dialysis machine, dialysis membrane, dialysis monitor, dialysis solution, dialysis technique, dialyzer, dialyzer, diffusion, elimination, elimination treatment, elimination treatment, end-stage kidney disease, end-stage renal disease, ESKD, ESRD, excrete, excretion, extra-body, extracorporeal, extracorporeal circuit, extracorporeal elimination, fibrinogen, fistula, fistulae, glycation, gradient, hemodiafiltration, hemodiafiltration, hemodialysis, hemofiltration, hemofiltration, hemoperfusion, hepatic support, hepatocytes, heterozygous, high-efficiency, high-volume, homeokinesis, homeostasis, homozygous, hydrophilization, hypercholesterolemia, immunoadsorption, immunoglobulins, intra-body, intracorporeal, intracorporeal elimination, kidney, kidney failure, kidney function, kidney functions, kidney transplantation, LDL-apheresis, lipids, lipoprotein, liver dialysis, liver support, liver transplantation, macroglobulin, MARS, membrane, membrane plasma separation, mid-dilution, high-flux, non-biologic liver support, OLT, orthotopic liver transplantation, particles, peritoneal dialysis, peritoneal membrane, peritoneum, permcath, physics principles, plasma, plasma proteins, plasmapheresis, postdilution, predilution, Prometheus, protein, purification, purification, renal failure, renal replacement, renal replacement treatment, semipermeable membrane, shorts, shunt, single pass albumin dialysis, SPAD, staphylococcal protein A, supportive therapy, synthetic graft, transplantation, UF, hemofiltration, ultracentrifugation, ultrafiltration, uremia, uremic toxins, vascular prosthesis, venous, venous-venous, water treatment

CONTENT

INTRODUCTION AND CLASSIFICATION

Blood purification methods are partial replacements for kidney function by adjusting the composition and properties of blood in extracorporeal (extra-body) circuit or circulation in dialyzer (hemofiltration, hemodiafiltration, and so on), i.e., extracorporeal elimination treatment (**ECET**) in the extracorporeal dialysis circuit.

We use the temporary non-tunneled or permanent tunneled hemodialysis catheters with cuffs to ensure enough blood flow. We introduce them through the internal jugular vein, subclavian vein, femoral vein, and rarely via the external jugular vein or inferior vena cava. Alternatively, we surgically create the arterial-venous fistulae (shunts, shorts) followed by arterialization of the blood vessel after the fistula, which, after formation, matures for 6-8 weeks before we can use it as vascular access for the extracorporeal elimination treatment (ECET).

The whole range of different methods that at least partially replace failed or failing renal (kidney) function is called Renal Replacement Therapy (**RRT**). Renal replacement therapy and extracorporeal (extra-body) elimination therapy are two mutually overlapping sets, with renal replacement therapy also including kidney transplantation, intracorporeal (intra-body) elimination treatment (PD = Peritoneal Dialysis), and the like in addition to extracorporeal elimination therapy. Methods of extracorporeal elimination therapy also include ways that cannot be unambiguously classified as RRT, since they also replace other organ functions or help to correct other pathophysiological disorders.

When talking about the primary, elimination function of the kidney, which aims to preserve the steadiness of the internal environment (homeostasis, or exactly homeokinesis), we can divide renal replacement therapy into three basic categories:

1. **Extracorporeal elimination treatment [ECET]**
2. **Intracorporeal elimination treatment [ICET]**
3. **Kidney transplantation from a living or dead donor (giver) [KTx or NTx]**

In addition to the three categories of renal replacement therapy (RRT) mentioned above, treatments are also being used to replace other kidney functions and complement the elimination methods of renal replacement therapy.

The detailed classification of the individual methods I base on the physics and chemical principles of treatment, the functions that the methodology can substitute, according to the vascular access, the dialysis solution used, or the type of therapy, substitution solutions, treatment regimens or modes and the like.

Here is the proposed classification as follows:

1) **EXTRACORPOREAL (EXTRA-BODY) ELIMINATION (EXCRETION) TREATMENT (THERAPY)**
   a) *Classification based on the basic physics and chemical principles of the treatment:*
      i) Methods mainly using only blood purification options that replace some kidney functions only
         (1) Hemodialysis
         (2) High-flux and high-efficiency hemodialysis
         (3) Isolated ("dry") ultrafiltration
         (4) Hemofiltration
            (a) Predilution
            (b) Postdilution
            (c) High-volume
         (5) Hemodiafiltration
            (a) Predilution
            (b) Mid-dilution hemodiafiltration
            (c) Postdilution
            (d) High-volume
      ii) Methods utilizing additional "enhanced" blood purification options and possibly replacing other functions of other organs detoxifying the body
         (1) Hemoperfusion
         (2) Membrane plasma separation (separation of plasma on the membrane)
         (3) Cascade filtration.
         (4) Immunoadsorption and apheresis.
         (5) Extracorporeal supportive treatment of the liver (liver dialysis)
         (6) Non-biological support of the liver.
            (a) PROMETHEUS system - system separating fractionated plasma
            (b) MARS system - molecular absorption recirculation system
            (c) SPAD – single pass albumin dialysis
         (7) Biological support of the liver (bio-artificial liver devices)

b) *Classification based on the duration:*
  (1) Intermittent (interrupted, discontinuous) methods
  (2) Continuous (continual, uninterrupted) means
c) *Classification based on vascular access:*
  (1) Arterial-venous methods
    (a) Catheterization of the central artery (most commonly femoral artery) and catheterization of the central vein
    (b) Catheterization of the central artery (most commonly femoral artery) and blood return to the peripheral vein
    (c) External arterial-venous graft
  (2) Venous-venous methods
    (a) Central venous catheter - non-tunneled catheter, without any cuff, acute
    (b) The permanent central venous catheter (permcath) – cuff-equipped tunneled catheter, chronic, long-lasting
    (c) Implantable port
    (d) Artificial artery-venous shunt followed by the arterialization of the venous system behind created short circuit - shunt (AV fistula)
    (e) Vascular prosthesis
      (i) Autologous (usually venous) graft.
      (ii) Synthetic graft.
d) *Classification based on the used dialysis and substitution solution:*
  (1) Bicarbonate method using bicarbonate solution (35 mmol/L of the bicarbonate and 3-5 mmol/L of the acetic acid)
  (2) Lactate method using the lactic acid solution
  (3) Acetate method using the acetic acid solution (38 mmol/L)
  (4) Citrate method using a citric acid solution

2) INTRACORPOREAL (INTRA-BODY) ELIMINATION (EXCRETION)
   TREATMENT (THERAPY)
   (1) **Intermittent peritoneal dialysis (IPD)**
   (2) **Continuous ambulatory/outpatient peritoneal dialysis (CAPD)**
   (3) **Automated peritoneal dialysis (APD)**
       (a) Night intermittent peritoneal dialysis (NIPD)
       (b) Continuous cyclic peritoneal dialysis (CCPD)
       (c) Optimized continuous peritoneal dialysis (OCPD) or PD Plus
       (d) Tidal peritoneal dialysis (TPD)
   (4) **Continuous flow peritoneal dialysis (CFPD)**

3) KIDNEY TRANSPLANTATION (KTX OR NTX) AS THE THIRD PILLAR
   OF THE RENAL REPLACING THERAPY (RRT)
   (1) **KTx from a living donor, relatives (blood or emotionally related)**
   (2) **KTx from a dead (cadaveric) donor (giver)**

HEMODIALYSIS, HEMOFILTRATION, AND HEMODIAFILTRATION

The fundamental prerequisite for the successful use of extracorporeal elimination therapy technology is the knowledge and successful application of several basic physics and chemical principles that we can describe as technological principles of extracorporeal elimination treatment.

These principles include:

A. Molecular diffusion.

B. Convection (membrane filtration).

C. Adsorption.

D. Osmosis (molecular diffusion of water).

BASIC PHYSICS AND CHEMICAL PRINCIPLES OF EXTRACORPOREAL ELIMINATION TREATMENT

Molecular diffusion, which is commonly called abbreviated merely diffusion, is the transfer of molecules from a higher concentration to the area of a lower level through random molecular motion.

Thus, diffusion is a spontaneous passive transport of a substance from a higher concentration environment to a lower concentration environment. Spread taking place through a semipermeable membrane is called dialysis. During hemodialysis, catabolites diffuse from the blood through the membrane into the dialysis solution and during this process they leave the body. The term back-diffusion refers to the passage of substances in the opposite direction, i.e., from the dialysis solution into the blood. It is used, for example, to correct acid-base imbalance (passing the essential molecule from the dialysis solution into the blood).

The semipermeable membrane permits the passage of substances of the specific molecular weight only. Contents whose molecular weight does not prevent passage through the semipermeable membrane go through it in the case of diffusion in the direction of the concentration gradient.

The term convection primary refers to the transfer of molecules in liquid environments and is a significant way of transferring heat and transferring substances. When using methods of extracorporeal elimination treatment, it is the transfer of materials by flow, namely the process of flooding of solutes together with the solvent through a semipermeable layer - membrane filtration. Solutions go through the coating through a process called filtration. Thus, it is the simultaneous transport of the solvent, in our case water and the solute through the sheet. Its driving force is in our case enough pressure gradient on the membrane.

Filtration is a mechanical or physical activity that uses a medium through which a fluid passes (e.g., a membrane), but a solid, eventually, to separate solids from liquids. Dissolved solutions do not pass through the medium. I should emphasize too that the separation is not complete and depends on the size and shape of the pores, the thickness of the medium as well as the mechanisms that occur during filtration.

The phenomenon used in methods of extracorporeal elimination treatment may be referred to as "sieving" as a single-layer membrane occurs as the filter medium. In the narrower sense, filtration refers to an event in which a multilayer medium occurs.

Ultrafiltration (UF) refers to membrane filtration using hydrostatic pressure on a semipermeable membrane. The solutes are retained on the layer, depending on their molecular weight, while water and some substances pass through the membrane.

In the case of membranes with hydrophobic properties, the phenomenon of adsorption uses the physics-chemical principles of the transfer of substances through the dialysis membrane. In some methods of extracorporeal elimination treatment, membrane adsorption significantly contributes to the total amount of material removed during the procedure.

Osmosis is the kind of water diffusion through a semipermeable membrane from a low concentration solute (high water potential) to a settlement with a high solute concentration (low water potential) in the solute concentration gradient.

It is a physical process in which the solvent transfers without energy input through a semipermeable membrane (solvent permeable but impermeable to solute), which separates two solutions with different concentrations.

Reverse osmosis is a high-pressure filtration through a very dense membrane. A wide range of undesirable aqueous impurities is retained both by a simple sieve effect and electrostatically too. In general, charged particles keep better than electrically neutral and multivalent ions better than monovalent cations and anions.

Dialysis is generally a process by which removes the nitrogenous (and other) waste products of metabolism, and the disorders of electrolyte, aqueous and acid-base balance associated with renal failure are corrected.

If you want to perform hemodialysis (HD), it is necessary to use a semipermeable membrane that allows the passage of water and solutes of lower molecular weight but does not release large molecules (e.g., proteins). For a better understanding, the urea molecular weight is 60 Daltons, 113 Daltons for creatinine, 1355 Daltons for vitamin B, 60,000 Daltons for albumin, and 140,000 Daltons for immunoglobulin IgG.

The extracorporeal circuit of hemodialysis consists of a dialyzer and a system of hoses, which bring blood into the dialyzer from the vascular access and return the purified blood to the patient. The dialysis solution (dialysate) is fed into the dialyzer by other hoses and then drained.

The term ultrafiltration (UF) refers to the convective flow of water and solutes dissolved in the direction of a pressure gradient caused by hydrostatic or osmotic forces. During hemodialysis, ultrafiltration is usually achieved by negative pressure on the compartment side of the dialyzer using a dialysate drainage pump (transmembrane pressure, abbreviated as "TMP"). The ultrafiltration rate depends on the pressure gradient and the type of dialysis membrane used.

Ultrafiltration is used during conventional hemodialysis merely to remove excess water accumulated between hemodialysis procedures by eating food, fluids, and metabolically formed pool, thus allowing us to balance the patient's intake and delivery balance and get rid of the accumulated water due to limited or complete lack of kidney ability to secrete urine in these patients. After counting the estimated amount of water lost in breathing, stool, and insensible perspiration (sweating) under normal circumstances and subtracting the metabolically produced water, we reach a value of about 650 mL. This amount together with the diuretic volume of a given patient becomes a springboard for us to calculate permitted intake fluid so that the patient does not exceed the inter-dialytic (from the end of the treatment to the beginning of the next procedure) weight gain of 2-3% (sometimes 4%) of his "dry" body weight.

The tactics of chronic dialysis therapy, as well as the frequency of dialysis, they all depend on the diuresis, metabolic and nutritional status of the patient and the currently established parameters of the adequacy of the dialysis treatment (e.g., determination of the Kt/V index). National Kidney Foundation Kidney Disease Outcomes Quality Initiative (NKF KDOQI)™ Guidelines [https://www.kidney.org/professionals/guidelines/guidelines_commentaries], Kidney Disease – Improving Global Outcomes (KDIGO) Guidelines [https://kdigo.org/guidelines/] and the European Renal Best Practice Guidelines (ERBP) [http://www.european-renal-best-practice.org/content/erbp-documents-topic] still recommend a standard three times a week 4-hour dialysis dose for all patients.

HEMOFILTRATION AND HEMODIAFILTRATION

Hemofiltration provides solute clearance solely through convection when the solutes are floated along with the solvent to flow through a semipermeable membrane downstream of an adequate pressure gradient. This process removes relatively high volumes of filtrate (approximately 40 liters per procedure). The substitute solution then replaces this amount.

Hemodiafiltration combines hemodialysis with high volumes of ultrafiltration comparing to the hemofiltration, i.e., it combines both convective and diffuse removal of renal retention solutes and other substances from the blood that passes through the semipermeable dialysis membrane.

The replacement fluid (replacement or substitution solution) must be ultrapure, with minimal endotoxin contamination as it is administered directly to the patient's blood. High permeable large membranes, high blood flow rates, and precise control of replacement volume are also required.

Hemofiltration provides better removal of substances of higher molecular weight (for example, β2-microglobulin, advanced glycation end products, and so on), improved clearance of uremic low molecular weight toxins and improved cardiovascular stability and blood pressure control over traditional intermittent hemodialysis.

DIALYSIS MEMBRANES

Classical dialysis membranes we divide into two groups:

A. Cellulose-based dialysis membranes.

B. Synthetic polymer dialysis membranes.

Cellulose membranes may cause complement and leukocyte activation, while plastic layers are characterized by higher biocompatibility in this regard. Unmodified cellulose membranes are low flow fluxes. The modified cellulosic membranes can be as low-flux as a high-flux one with higher (cellulose triacetate) or lower (cellulose acetate) biocompatibility. Cellulose-based dialysis membranes include non-modified cellulose dialysis membranes, regenerated cellulose dialysis membranes, and synthetically modified membranes by chemically changing cellobiose.

A second large group of dialysis membranes is the group of dialysis membranes of synthetic polymers. In their use, a higher β2-microglobulin clearance was found compared to cellulose membranes with the same solute clearance. The various hydrophilization methods create these types of layers. These include polysulfone, polyacrylonitrile, and polyamide. They are hydrophobic and therefore must be done hydrophilic to use them as a filter for blood toxins. Only the ethyl vinyl alcohol copolymers are hydrophilic so that they utilize without modification. For hemofiltration (either continuous or high flow) and related methods, we use synthetic membranes only.

DIALYZERS

The dialyzer (also called a filter) consists of a rigid housing usually made of polyurethane in which hollow fibers form capillaries or parallel plates made of a dialysis membrane. Furthermore, it has two inlets for infiltration and leakage of blood and another two inlets for circulation of the dialysis solution. Capillaries or parallel plates allow maximizing the area of the dialysis membrane that encounters blood and dialysis solution. Other techniques, as well as nanotechnologies for aligning the capillaries in the dialyzer, are used to assemble the newer dialyzers so that the effectiveness of membrane surface contact with the blood and dialysis solution we further increase. In capillary dialyzers, the blood flows through the inside of the hollow fibers (inside the capillaries), and in the so-called, the plate dialyzers the blood flows alternately between the individual plate layers of the dialysis membrane.

Capillary dialyzers have a slightly smaller fill volume and can more easily retain ethylene oxide (when used as a sterilizing agent), while a lesser risk of blood coagulation in the dialyzer we prefer for plate dialyzers. Currently, capillary dialyzers we use most commonly in all countries due to their higher efficiency.

DIALYSIS DEVICE (MONITOR, MACHINE, APPARATUS)

Dialysis devices, sometimes also called dialysis monitors, basically consist of several essential parts, which are:

a) The blood pump, usually peristaltic.

b) Air detector.

c) A system for administering heparin or administering other anticoagulation.

d) Dialysate preparation system.

e) Ultrafiltration control.

f) Sodium profiling.

g) Additional water and/or dialysate ultrafilters.

h) Automatic chemical and thermal disinfection.

i) Single-needle dialysis (S/N HD) or two-needle dialysis (D/N HD) mechanisms.

j) Pressure detectors.

k) Blood leak detector.

l) Detection of blood present in extracorporeal circulation (circuit).

m) More modern devices also include individual monitors to calculate and monitor Kt/V index in real-time settings, automatic blood pressure monitoring and/or ECG, blood volume monitors, current oxygen saturation monitors, fluid balance monitors, and patient hydration, recirculation measurement and the like.

DIALYSATE (DIALYSIS SOLUTION)

Typically, the dialysis solutions are prepared from concentrates and contain either acetate, citrate or bicarbonate as the buffer system. Separate acetate is currently rarely used. The exact composition we can adjust as necessary, and the use of individualized dialysis prescription for the patient is increased, resulting in increased requirements for the dialysis center logistics. Modern dialysis devices already allow accurate preparation of the dialysis solution and monitor its composition by conductivity measurement. The second option is to centrally prepare the dialysis solution from the concentrates in the dialysis center and distribute the already prepared dialysis solutions to the individual dialysis devices. However, central preparation does not allow individualization of dialysis solutions for individual patients.

For the preparation of dialysis solutions, treated water is required to be free of almost all impurities. We prepare it in water treatment devices. The initial treatment phase is characterized by filtration (gravel filter of coarse contaminants, carbon filter, deionization filter, and others), while reverse osmosis we use in the second phase.

CONTINUOUS RENAL REPLACEMENT THERAPY (CRRT)

Continuous Renal Replacement Therapy (CRRT) is appropriate in cases of hemodynamically significantly compromised patients with acute renal failure (AKI = Acute Kidney Injury). They allow slow and gentle removal of solutes and fluids while avoiding massive shifts of intravascular fluid and minimizing electrolyte disturbances, hypotension, and arrhythmias. Hypotension that occurs during conventional intermittent hemodialysis may contribute to further ischemic attacks on the kidneys afflicted with AKI, disrupting the healing and restoration process. The uremia ceases better at CRRT than at intermittent hemodialysis (iHD) in catabolic AKI patients. Ultrafiltration we can achieve either continuously or as needed to ensure the need to maintain fluid balance in the patient, where parenteral and enteral nutrition and intravenous administration are usually required. Therapeutic drug levels we can manage more reliably during CRRT. It is possible to continuously remove inflammatory mediators, which contributes to better hemodynamic stability.

COMPLICATIONS OF EXTRACORPOREAL ELIMINATION TREATMENT

Acute complications of the extracorporeal elimination treatment (ECET) include hypotension, muscle cramps, disequilibrium syndrome, electrolyte disturbances, severe allergic reactions, fever, headache, hypertension, air embolism, hemolysis, bleeding episodes, arrhythmias and blood clotting in extracorporeal circulation.

Chronic ECET complications are most often due to the imperfect replacement of healthy kidney function, and cardiovascular, metabolic, urological and neurological complications, including psychological and psychiatric difficulties often associated with impaired adaptation to long-term dialysis therapy, are the most significant.

PERITONEAL DIALYSIS

Peritoneal dialysis is a method of treating chronic renal failure, that is, one of the renal replacement therapy (RRT) methods, a renal replacement therapy that is now generally considered to be utterly comparable to hemodialysis and other related RRT methods.

In Slovakia, the number of peritoneal dialysis patients currently account for approximately 5.3% of all patients requiring regular dialysis. In the Czech Republic, 8.4% of patients treated with PD in 2009. In some countries, RRT significantly treats more patients, such as 36% in Canada, 41.9% in Australia and even 85% in Mexico. In Europe, this figure usually is between 2 and 10%.

WHY CHOOSE PERITONEAL DIALYSIS

In an integrated patient care system for chronic renal failure, we should prefer the peritoneal dialysis (PD) as a first-choice method for initiating first-choice treatment. The main reasons include prolonged retention of residual diuresis (longer survival in the first two years), continuous ultrafiltration and catabolite removal, less risk of hepatitis transmission, HIV, and protection of the vascular system for the period when vascular access for hemodialysis is necessary. Patients have lower mortality when treated first with peritoneal dialysis followed by hemodialysis as opposed to, and the first method of treatment is hemodialysis.

PERITONEAL DIALYSIS BASIC PRINCIPLES

Peritoneal dialysis we based on the removal of metabolites and the adjustment of the internal environment on the principle of substance exchange between blood and peritoneal dialysis solution, which we impregnate into the peritoneal (abdominal) cavity. The transfer of substances takes place via the peritoneum, which is a barrier between the blood circulation and the peritoneal cavity.

From this point of view, the peritoneum consists of three layers. A mesothelium - a flatlining composed of mesothelial cells - is located on the surface towards the abdominal cavity. There is an interstitial tissue beneath the mesothelium - an intermediate layer of fabric. In the interstitial tissue, capillaries are running whose wall is separated from the mesothelium by this nested tissue. The third layer of the peritoneal dialysis membrane is the endothelial lining of the individual capillaries along with the basement membrane of this endothelium.

The transport of individual substances through the peritoneal dialysis membrane (mesothelium, interstitial tissue, endothelium basement membrane) we base on two basic physics and chemical principles: diffusion and convection. Water removal is through osmosis.

Thus, the peritoneal dialysis solution must contain an osmotically active substance we achieve an osmotic gradient. The osmotically active material is usually glucose, but answers with other osmotically active elements such as glucose polymer (icodextrin) we used too. Solutions with three different glucose concentrations are commonly available, which are also color-coded on the packaging (e.g., yellow, green, and red solutions). These are glucose solutions of 1.36% (1.5%), 2.27% (2.5%) and 3.86% (4.25%) concentrations I show in parentheses after conversion to the currently used glucose monohydrate.

Metabolic acidosis in patients with chronic renal failure at the ESRD stage and the need for renal replacement therapy can be corrected for peritoneal dialysis by addition of a base to the peritoneal dialysis solution. Due to the instability of sodium bicarbonate and the precipitation of calcium and magnesium salts in the solution, lactate is usually used, from which bicarbonate is formed metabolically in the liver.

Not a significant amount of protein passing through the peritoneal dialysis membrane, representing daily losses of about 10 grams, is dependent upon the characteristics of the peritoneum of the patient. With higher peritoneum permeability, protein losses are also higher.

LONG-TERM PERITONEAL DIALYSIS

During long-term peritoneal dialysis, the peritoneum changes morphologically and functionally. There are degeneration and desquamation of mesothelial cells, thickening and fibrotic changes of the interstitial tissue, and proliferation of vessels with concomitant hyalinization of the vascular wall and thickening of the endothelium. From a functional point of view, the ultrafiltration capability loses due to the too high permeability of the peritoneum.

PERITONEAL DIALYSIS IN PRACTICE

A peritoneal dialysis catheter is used to provide access to the abdominal cavity.

Peritoneal dialysis can be carried out in two primary ways, either manually in continuous ambulatory peritoneal dialysis (CAPD) mode, or by a cyclic peritoneal dialysis exchange device, so-called "cycler" in automated peritoneal dialysis (APD) mode. Different PD regimens we can classify into chronic peritoneal dialysis based on the schedule of exchanges.

An irreplaceable and substantial role in the success of PD application is the education of the patient, which we put mainly on the dialysis nurse's shoulders

PERITONEAL DIALYSIS COMPLICATIONS

The most severe complications of peritoneal dialysis therapy are infectious complications, including, but not limited to, acute peritonitis (inflammation of the peritoneal catheter) and infections along the peritoneal dialysis catheter (tunnel infections).

Non-infectious complications of PD include difficulties associated with peritoneal dialysis catheter (leak, occlusion, dislocation, cuff release, intraperitoneal decubitus necrosis), complications related to increased intraperitoneal pressure (hernia, lumbago, hydrothorax, pelvic organ prolapse), disturbances in water and electrolyte , metabolic complications (malnutrition, lipoproteinemia disorders, hyperglycemia), hemoperitoneum, abdominal pain, organ gastrointestinal and respiratory complications, pneumoperitoneum, disorders of ultrafiltration and technical difficulties.

PERITONEAL DIALYSIS ADEQUACY

The assessment of adequacy of peritoneal dialysis includes evaluation of patient clinical status, biochemical examinations, hydration and nutritional status, ultrafiltration size, kinetic modeling of urea, creatinine and sodium removal for the patient (Twardovski's [PET] peritoneal equilibration test and its modification, weekly determination of the creatinine clearance and Kt/V index). An adequately dialyzed patient does not have subjective complaints, has a healthy appetite, a stable weight, and has no hypertension. However, polymorphic patients have an inferior prognosis regardless of the quality of the dialysis treatment.

Part of the comprehensive treatment of the patient with peritoneal dialysis (as well as hemodialysis) is the treatment of renal anemia and mineral bone disease in the impairment of phosphorus/phosphates and calcium metabolism as well as the treatment of lipoproteinemia disorders and the preparation of patients for kidney transplantation.

LIVER DIALYSIS - ARTIFICIAL DETOXIFICATION HEPATIC SUPPORTIVE THERAPY

Since the 1950s, some methodologies have been used to help the failing liver. It was a variety of therapies ranging from drug treatment regimens to liver support devices and liver transplantation. Currently, the standard treatment for acute liver failure (ALF) is orthotopic liver transplantation (OLT = Orthotopic Liver Transplantation).

Due to the high mortality rates and prolonged waiting times for transplantation, the interest in techniques that allow temporary support of the liver function is revived to overcome the period when a patient with acute liver failure (ALF) waits for OLT or liver regeneration. In general, these techniques we can divide into two primary groups, namely non-biologic and biologic liver support.

Usually, hemodialysis is used in renal failure but has limited use in liver failure since it does not remove albumin-bound toxins. The most promising non-biological supportive therapies combine the detoxification of water-soluble and protein-bound toxins in a dialysis system.

Biological approaches rely on liver or hepatocyte functions of xenogeneic or human origin, which can be used to support the patient's liver. These functions include detoxification, several metabolic functions, and the synthesis of proteins and other molecules.

Isolated liver cells we used in various configurations: suspended, attached to the substrate, and encapsulated in semipermeable membranes. Hepatocytes used to support the liver can be divided into two categories: implantable systems and extracorporeal systems.

Bioartificial liver systems consist of an artificial component, i. the bioreactor and its equipment and the biocomponent, i.e., hepatocytes. Currently, there is a significant increase and development of various bio-functional hepatic systems, in practice, so far 11 different devices have been used.

OTHER METHODS OF EXTRACORPOREAL ELIMINATION TREATMENT

Other important methods of extracorporeal elimination therapy include plasmapheresis, which can be performed either by ultracentrifugation or in the form of membrane separation of plasma (MPS = Membrane Plasma Separation). During MPS, separated plasma can be further treated to remove certain types of substances, for example, by immunoadsorption, and thus processed can be returned to the patient. Plasma therapy widely uses in the treatment of various autoimmune diseases.

Immunoadsorption devices we can divide into non-selective, semi-selective, and highly selective adsorbers. Non-selective adsorbers (dextran sulfate, tryptophan, and phenylalanine) reduce plasma levels of many different agents such as fibrinogen, albumin, lipids, and immunoglobulins. Semiselective adsorbers (staphylococcal protein A, anti-human Ig adsorber) show an affinity for only one group of plasma proteins. High-selective adsorbers eliminate specific substances without altering blood levels of other plasma components.

Another of the existing methods of extracorporeal elimination treatment is LDL-apheresis, a form of apheresis that mimics the dialysis technique designed to eliminate low-density lipoprotein particles containing cholesterol (LDL-cholesterol). It is used in rare homozygous familial hypercholesterolemia, in its heterozygous form if it does not deal with routine medical treatment and similar diseases.

BIBLIOGRAPHY

Abu-Aisha, H. & Elamin, S., 2010. PERITONEAL DIALYSIS IN AFRICA. *Peritoneal Dialysis International,* 30(1), pp. 23-28.

Agar, J., 2010. Review: understanding sorbent dialysis systems. *Nephrology,* 15(4), pp. 406-411.

Alexander, R. T. et al., 2012. Kidney stones and kidney function loss: a cohort study. *BMJ,* 345(), p.

Am, S. et al., 2004. *Peritoneal dialysis in end-stage renal disease after liver transplantation..* [Online]
Available at: http://ncbi.nlm.nih.gov/pubmed/15384804
[Accessed 17 3 2019].

Anon., *Amyloidosis and Kidney Disease.* [Online]
Available at: http://kidney.niddk.nih.gov/kudiseases/pubs/amyloidosis/
[Accessed 17 3 2019].

Anon., *Atlas of Diseases of the Kidney, Volume 5, Principles of Dialysis: Diffusion, Convection, and Dialysis Machines.* [Online]
Available at: http://www.kidneyatlas.org/book5/adk5-01.ccc.QXD.pdf
[Accessed 17 3 2019].

Anon., *Kidney Disease Improving Global Outcomes (KDIGO).* [Online]
Available at: http://kdigo.org/home/
[Accessed 17 3 2019].

Anon., *Kidney Overview.* [Online]
Available at: http://www.webmd.com/a-to-z-guides/function-kidneys?page=4#1
[Accessed 17 3 2019].

Anon., *Kidney Transplant.* [Online]
Available at: http://www.nhs.uk/conditions/Kidney-transplant/Pages/Introduction.aspx
[Accessed 17 3 2019].

Anon., *Kidney transplant: MedlinePlus Medical Encyclopedia.* [Online]
Available at:
https://www.nlm.nih.gov/medlineplus/ency/article/003005.htm
[Accessed 17 3 2019].

Anon., *National Kidney Registry.* [Online]
Available at: http://www.kidneyregistry.org/?cookie=1
[Accessed 17 3 2019].

Anon., *Polycystic kidney disease.* [Online]
Available at: http://ghr.nlm.nih.gov/condition/polycystic-kidney-disease
[Accessed 17 3 2019].

Anon., *Printing a human kidney.* [Online]
Available at:
http://www.ted.com/talks/anthony_atala_printing_a_human_kidney.ht
ml
[Accessed 17 3 2019].

Anon., *The Kidneys and How They Work.* [Online]
Available at: http://www.niddk.nih.gov/health-information/health-
topics/Anatomy/kidneys-how-they-work/Pages/anatomy.aspx
[Accessed 17 3 2019].

Baboolal, K. et al., 2008. The cost of renal dialysis in a UK setting—a
multicentre study. *Nephrology Dialysis Transplantation,* 23(6), pp.
1982-1989.

Bagshaw, S. M. & Wald, R., 2011. Renal Replacement Therapy: When to
Start. *Contributions To Nephrology,* 174(), pp. 232-241.

Bajaj, P., 2008. Renal Replacement Therapy. *Indian Journal of
Anaesthesia,* 52(6), p. 753.

Bargman, J. M., 2007. New technologies in peritoneal dialysis. *Clinical
Journal of The American Society of Nephrology,* 2(3), pp. 576-580.

Berger, J. R. & Hedayati, S. S., 2012. Renal Replacement Therapy in the
Elderly Population. *Clinical Journal of The American Society of
Nephrology,* 7(6), pp. 1039-1046.

Birmelé, B. et al., 2004. Death after withdrawal from dialysis: the most common cause of death in a French dialysis population. *Nephrology Dialysis Transplantation,* 19(3), pp. 686-691.

Bray, B. D. et al., 2014. How safe is renal replacement therapy? A national study of mortality and adverse events contributing to the death of renal replacement therapy recipients. *Nephrology Dialysis Transplantation,* 29(3), pp. 681-687.

Coresh, J., 2012. A decade after the KDOQI CKD guidelines: impact on research. *American Journal of Kidney Diseases,* 60(5), pp. 701-704.

Cruz, D. N. et al., 2012. Renal Replacement Therapies for Prevention of Radiocontrast-induced Nephropathy: A Systematic Review. *The American Journal of Medicine,* 125(1), pp. 66-78.

Daugirdas, J. T., 2013. Dialysis time, survival, and dose-targeting bias. *Kidney International,* 83(1), pp. 9-13.

Debowska, M., Lindholm, B. & Waniewski, J., 2011. *Kinetic Modeling and Adequacy of Dialysis.* [Online]
Available at: http://cdn.intechopen.com/pdfs/21269.pdf
[Accessed 17 3 2019].

Deepa, C. & Muralidhar, K., 2012. Renal replacement therapy in ICU. *Journal of Anaesthesiology Clinical Pharmacology,* 28(3), pp. 386-396.

Deray, G., 2006. Dialysis and iodinated contrast media. *Kidney International,* 69(100), p.

Dirkes, S. & Hodge, K., 2007. Continuous Renal Replacement Therapy in the Adult Intensive Care Unit: History and Current Trends. *Critical Care Nurse,*27(2), pp. 61-80.

Eissa, M. A. et al., 2010. Factors Affecting Hemodialysis Patients' Satisfaction with Their Dialysis Therapy. *International Journal of Nephrology,* 2010(), pp. 342901-342901.

Fan, S., 2005. *Use of MARS dialysis in patients with liver failure in Hong Kong.* [Online]

Available at: http://hub.hku.hk/handle/10722/108156
[Accessed 17 3 2019].

Fasolo, L., Rocha, L., Campbell, S. & Peixoto, A. J., 2006. Diagnostic relevance of pyuria in dialysis patients. *Kidney International,* 70(11), pp. 2035-2038.

Fissell, W. H., Fleischman, A. J., Humes, H. D. & Roy, S., 2007. Development of continuous implantable renal replacement: past and future. *Translational Research,* 150(6), pp. 327-336.

Flieg, R., Aldinger, S., Storr, M. & Krause, B., 2013. *Liver support system.* [Online]
Available at: http://freepatentsonline.com/y2015/0273127.html
[Accessed 17 3 2019].

Foster, M. C. et al., 2011. Fatty Kidney, Hypertension, and Chronic Kidney Disease The Framingham Heart Study. *Hypertension,* 58(5), pp. 784-790.

Galbusera, M., Remuzzi, G. & Boccardo, P., 2009. Treatment of Bleeding in Dialysis Patients. *Seminars in Dialysis,* 22(3), pp. 279-286.

Gallieni, M., Saxena, R. & Davidson, I., 2009. Dialysis access in Europe and North America: are we on the same path?. *Seminars in Interventional Radiology,* 26(2), pp. 96-105.

Grinsted, D. P., *Kidney failure (renal failure with uremia, or azotemia).* [Online]
Available at:
http://www.netdoctor.co.uk/diseases/facts/kidneyfailure.htm
[Accessed 17 3 2019].

Griva, K. et al., 2014. Non-Adherence in Patients on Peritoneal Dialysis: A Systematic Review. *PLOS ONE,* 9(2), p.

Hall, N. A. & Fox, A., 2006. Renal replacement therapies in critical care. *Continuing Education in Anaesthesia, Critical Care & Pain,* 6(5), pp. 197-202.

Hartmann, A. et al., 2003. The risk of living kidney donation. *Nephrology Dialysis Transplantation,* 18(5), pp. 871-873.

Held, P. J., Garcia, J. R., Pauly, M. V. & Cahn, M. A., 1990. Price of Dialysis, Unit Staffing, and Length of Dialysis Treatments. *American Journal of Kidney Diseases,* 15(5), pp. 441-450.

Honore, P. M. et al., 2013. Con: Dialy- and continuous renal replacement (CRRT) trauma during renal replacement therapy: still under-recognized but on the way to better diagnostic understanding and prevention. *Nephrology Dialysis Transplantation,* 28(11), pp. 2723-2728.

Hoste, E., Hoste, E. & Dhondt, A., 2011. Clinical review: Use of renal replacement therapies in special groups of ICU patients. *Critical Care,* 16(1), pp. 201-201.

Hou, S., 2008. Pregnancy in Women on Dialysis: Is Success a Matter of Time?. *Clinical Journal of The American Society of Nephrology,* 3(2), pp. 312-313.

Chaudhary, K., Sangha, H. & Khanna, R., 2011. Peritoneal Dialysis First: Rationale. *Clinical Journal of The American Society of Nephrology,* 6(2), pp. 447-456.

Chow, K. M. et al., 2006. Predictive Value of Dialysate Cell Counts in Peritonitis Complicating Peritoneal Dialysis. *Clinical Journal of The American Society of Nephrology,* 1(4), pp. 768-773.

Ito, M. et al., 2013. Peritoneal dialysis - A. *Nephrology Dialysis Transplantation,* 28(), p.

Jaar, B. G. et al., 2009. Timing, causes, predictors, and prognosis of switching from peritoneal dialysis to hemodialysis: a prospective study. *BMC Nephrology,* 10(1), pp. 3-3.

Jacobs, C., 2000. At which stage of renal failure should dialysis be started. *Nephrology Dialysis Transplantation,* 15(3), pp. 305-307.

John, S. & Eckardt, K.-U., 2007. Renal Replacement Strategies in the ICU. *Chest,* 132(4), pp. 1379-1388.

Joo, D. J. et al., 2012. *Renal Replacement Therapy: Available Information Versus Demands of Patients.* [Online]
Available at:
https://sciencedirect.com/science/article/pii/s0041134511017131#!
[Accessed 17 3 2019].

Kalirao, P. et al., 2011. Cognitive impairment in peritoneal dialysis patients. *American Journal of Kidney Diseases,* 57(4), pp. 612-620.

Kim, Y.-J.et al., 2005. The effect of dialysis needle size on hemodialysis adequacy. *Hemodialysis International,* 9(1), pp. 76-76.

Kliger, A. S. & Finkelstein, F. O., 2003. Which patients choose to stop dialysis. *Nephrology Dialysis Transplantation,* 18(5), pp. 869-871.

K, O., 2003. Acute adverse effects of dialysis. *Vnitrˇní lékarˇství,* , 49(2), p. 134.

Krivoshiev, S. et al., 1989. Termination of Dialysis Treatment. *Nephrology Dialysis Transplantation,* 4(6), pp. 602-602.

Leblanc, M., Ouimet, D. & Pichette, V., 2008. Dialysate Leaks in Peritoneal Dialysis. *Seminars in Dialysis,* 14(1), pp. 50-54.

Locatelli, F. et al., 2005. Dialysis dose and frequency. *Nephrology Dialysis Transplantation,* 20(2), pp. 285-296.

Lo, W. K. et al., 2008. PREPARING PATIENTS FOR PERITONEAL DIALYSIS. *Peritoneal Dialysis International,* 28(), p.

Luckritz, K. E. & Symons, J. M., 2009. *Renal Replacement Therapy in the ICU.* [Online]
Available at: https://link.springer.com/chapter/10.1007/978-3-540-74425-2_8
[Accessed 17 3 2019].

Macedo, E. & Mehta, R. L., 2010. Early vs late start of dialysis: it's all about timing. *Critical Care,* 14(1), pp. 112-112.

Mahadeshwar, T., Kim, H., Tikotekar, A. & Parikh, A., 2013. The timing of renal replacement therapy: is it when or how much?. *Critical Care,* 17(4), pp. 445-445.

McCauley, J., Gaynord, M., Hrinya, M. & Starzl, T. E., 1993. *Dialysis in Liver Failure and Liver Transplantation.* [Online]
Available at: https://ncbi.nlm.nih.gov/pmc/articles/pmc2954670
[Accessed 17 3 2019].

Metcalfe, W. et al., 2002. Acute renal failure requiring renal replacement therapy: incidence and outcome. *QJM: An International Journal of Medicine,* 95(9), pp. 579-583.

Mjøen, G. et al., 2014. Long-term risks for kidney donors. *Kidney International,* 86(1), pp. 162-167.

Mogyorosy, Z., Mucsi, I. & Rosivall, L., 2003. Renal replacement therapy in Hungary: the decade of transition. *Nephrology Dialysis Transplantation,* 18(6), pp. 1066-1071.

Muzaale, A. D. et al., 2014. Risk of End-Stage Renal Disease Following Live Kidney Donation. *JAMA,* 311(6), pp. 579-586.

Neovius, M. et al., 2014. Mortality in chronic kidney disease and renal replacement therapy: a population-based cohort study. *BMJ Open,* 4(2), p.

Noordzij, M. & Jager, K. J., 2012. Survival comparisons between hemodialysis and peritoneal dialysis. *Nephrology Dialysis Transplantation,* 27(9), pp. 3385-3387.

Palatnik, L., *A Kidney To Give: Why I donated my kidney to someone, I didn't know.* [Online]
Available at: http://www.aish.com/sp/so/48937647.html#
[Accessed 17 3 2019].

Palevsky, P. M., 2005. Renal Replacement Therapy I: Indications and Timing. *Critical Care Clinics,* 21(2), pp. 347-356.

Palevsky, P. M., 2013. Renal Replacement Therapy in Acute Kidney Injury. *Advances in Chronic Kidney Disease,* 20(1), pp. 76-84.

Pannu, N. & Gibney, R. T. N., 2005. Renal replacement therapy in the intensive care unit. *Therapeutics and Clinical Risk Management,* 1(2), pp. 141-150.

Perkovic, V., 2013. *KDIGO Blood Pressure Guideline Presentation.*
[Online]
Available at: http://georgeinstitute.org/publications/kdigo-blood-pressure-guideline-presentation
[Accessed 17 3 2019].

Perl, J. et al., 2011. Impact of Dialysis Modality on Survival after Kidney Transplant Failure. *Clinical Journal of The American Society of Nephrology,* 6(3), pp. 582-590.

Prins, K. W., Wille, K. M., Tallaj, J. A. & Tolwani, A., 2015. Assessing continuous renal replacement therapy as a rescue strategy in cardiorenal syndrome 1. *NDT Plus,* 8(1), pp. 87-92.

Rabindranath, K. S., Adams, J., MacLeod, A. M. & Muirhead, N., 2007. Intermittent versus continuous renal replacement therapy for acute renal failure in adults. *Cochrane Database of Systematic Reviews,* (3), p.

Rees, L., 2007. LONG-TERM PERITONEAL DIALYSIS IN INFANTS. *Peritoneal Dialysis International,* 27(), p.

Rj, M. et al., 2011. Factors Affecting Employment at Initiation of Dialysis. *Clinical Journal of The American Society of Nephrology,* 6(3), pp. 489-496.

Robinski, M. et al., 2014. The Choice of Renal Replacement Therapy (CORETH) project: study design and methods. *NDT Plus,* 7(6), pp. 575-581.

Romagnani, P., Romagnani, P. & Kalluri, R., 2009. Possible mechanisms of kidney repair. *Fibrogenesis & Tissue Repair,* , 2(1), pp. 3-3.

Ronco, C. & Bellomo, R., 1996. Complications with continuous renal replacement therapy. *American Journal of Kidney Diseases,* 28(5), p.

Ronco, C. et al., 2001. Machines for Continuous Renal Replacement Therapy. *Contributions To Nephrology,* 132(132), pp. 323-334.

Ronco, C. & Ricci, Z., 2008. Renal replacement therapies: physiological review. *Intensive Care Medicine,* , 34(12), pp. 2139-2146.

Rosansky, S. J., Glassock, R. J. & Clark, W. F., 2011. Early start of dialysis: a critical review. *Clinical Journal of The American Society of Nephrology,* 6(5), pp. 1222-1228.

Salizzoni, M. et al., 2004. *Sequential liver–kidney transplantation.* [Online]
Available at:
https://sciencedirect.com/science/article/pii/s0041134504001721
[Accessed 17 3 2019].

Sandhu, J., 2002. Dialysis Ports: A New Totally Implantable Option for Hemodialysis Access. *Techniques in Vascular and Interventional Radiology,* 5(2), pp. 108-113.

Santoro, A. & Guadagni, G., 2010. Dialysis membrane: from convection to adsorption. *NDT Plus,* 3(), p.

Sarkar, S., 2008. Continuous Renal Replacement Therapy (CRRT). *The Internet Journal of Anesthesiology,* 21(1), p.

Shapiro, E., Goldfarb, D. A. & Ritchey, M. L., 2003. The Congenital and Acquired Solitary Kidney. *Reviews in urology,* 5(1), p. 2.

Shroff, R. & Ledermann, S. E., 2006. Long-term outcome of chronic dialysis in children. *Pediatric Nephrology,* 24(3), pp. 463-474.

Singh, H. K. & Nickeleit, V., 2004. Kidney disease caused by viral infections. *Current Diagnostic Pathology,* 10(1), pp. 11-21.

Sinnakirouchenan, R. & Holley, J. L., 2011. Peritoneal dialysis versus hemodialysis: Risks, benefits, and access issues. *Advances in Chronic Kidney Disease,* 18(6), pp. 428-432.

Smeets, E. et al., 2003. Prevention of biofilm formation in dialysis water treatment systems. *Kidney International,* 63(4), pp. 1574-1576.

Smyth, A., 2012. End-Stage Renal Disease and Renal Replacement Therapy in Older Patients. *Nephro-urology monthly,* 4(2), pp. 425-430.

Solez, K., 2005. Web Sites of Interest—KDIGO: www.kdigo.org. *Advances in Chronic Kidney Disease,* 12(2), p. 243.

Stack, A. G. & Messana, J. M., 2000. Renal Replacement Therapy in the Elderly: Medical, Ethical, and Psychosocial Considerations. *Advances in Renal Replacement Therapy,* 7(1), pp. 52-62.

Stanley, M., 2010. Peritoneal dialysis versus hemodialysis (adult). *Nephrology,* 15(), p.

Su, Z., 2013. *Peritoneal Dialysis Catheter Placement and Management.* [Online]
Available at: https://intechopen.com/books/the-latest-in-peritoneal-dialysis/peritoneal-dialysis-catheter-placement-and-management
[Accessed 17 3 2019].

Tangri, N. et al., 2011. A Predictive Model for the Progression of Chronic Kidney Disease to Kidney Failure. *JAMA,* 305(15), pp. 1553-1559.

Tarlo, S. M., 2003. Peritoneal dialysis and cough. *Peritoneal Dialysis International,* 23(5), pp. 424-426.

Tattersall, J. et al., 2011. When to start dialysis: updated guidance following publication of the Initiating Dialysis Early and Late (IDEAL) study. *Nephrology Dialysis Transplantation,* 26(7), pp. 2082-2086.

Termorshuizen, F. et al., 2003. Hemodialysis and Peritoneal Dialysis: Comparison of Adjusted Mortality Rates According to the Duration of Dialysis: Analysis of the Netherlands Cooperative Study on the Adequacy of Dialysis 2. *Journal of The American Society of Nephrology,* 14(11), pp. 2851-2860.

Tokgoz, B., 2009. CLINICAL ADVANTAGES OF PERITONEAL DIALYSIS. *Peritoneal Dialysis International,* 29(), p.

White, C. A., Pilkey, R. M., Lam, M. & Holland, D., 2002. Pre-dialysis clinic attendance improves quality of life among hemodialysis patients. *BMC Nephrology,* 3(1), pp. 3-3.

Wühl, E. et al., 2014. Renal replacement therapy for rare diseases affecting the kidney: an analysis of the ERA-EDTA Registry. *Nephrology Dialysis Transplantation,* 29(), p.

Yee, J., 2008. Diabetic Kidney Disease: Chronic Kidney Disease and Diabetes. *Diabetes Spectrum,* 21(1), pp. 8-10.

This topic in more detail and like you can find in my publications from my
Kidney Replacement series
published on Amazon – Kindle Direct Publishing, e.g.,

BLOOD PURIFICATION

Specialized Work

By

Lubomir POLASCIN, MD

On

EXTRACORPOREAL ELIMINATION TREATMENT

Dialysis interventions to achieve required blood composition changes in men by its artificial machine purification on the principles of diffusion/dialysis, convection (membrane filtration), adsorption and osmosis.

The End

www.ingramcontent.com/pod-product-compliance
Lightning Source LLC
Chambersburg PA
CBHW021925170526
45157CB00005B/2186